June 2024

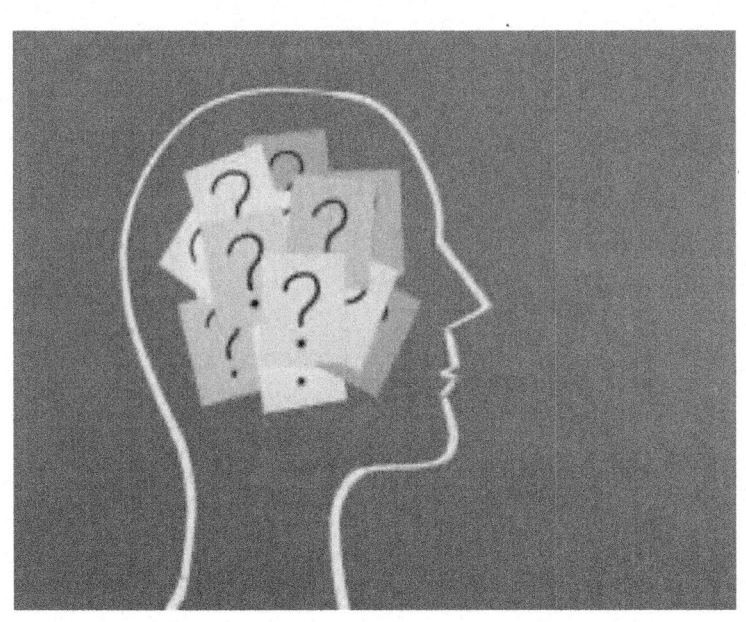

ACHIEVING YOUR BEST BRAIN HEALTH WITH MILD COGNITIVE IMPAIRMENT

Kari Herman, BSN, RN-BC

Copyright © 2022 Kari Herman

All rights reserved. No part of this book may be copied or reproduced in any form without permission in writing from the publisher except by a reviewer who may quote brief passages for review purposes.

TABLE OF CONTENTS

INTRODUCTION 1

CHAPTER ONE   BRAIN BASICS 3
- Cerebellum 3
- Brain Stem 4
- Cerebrum 4
- The Four Lobes of the Brain 5
- Cerebral Cortex 8
- The Hippocampi 9
- Neurons 9
- Blood Supply Network 10

CHAPTER TWO   MEMORY PROCESSING 11
- Stages of Memory 11
- Memory Testing 11
- Normal Age-Related Changes 12
- Reversible Causes of Memory Impairment 14

CHAPTER THREE   MILD COGNITIVE IMPAIRMENT 17
- Types of MCI 18
- Possible Causes of MCI 19
- Prognosis 24

CHAPTER FOUR   MCI AND MILD DEMENTIA CAUSED BY ALZHEIMER'S DISEASE 27
- Vascular Dementia 30
- Lewy Body Dementia 32
- Frontotemporal Dementia 34

CHAPTER FIVE   WHY I SHOULD PAY ATTENTION 37
- Benefits of an Early Diagnosis 37
- Working with Your Doctor 38
- Getting Ready for a Doctor's Appointment 39
- How a Diagnosis is Made 40
- Specialists 40

CHAPTER SIX   HOW WILL I GO ON? 43
- Adjusting to a New Diagnosis 43
- Coping 44

CHAPTER SEVEN   HOW WILL THE ROLES IN MY LIFE CHANGE? 47
- Changes 47
- Caregiver Wellness 49

CHAPTER EIGHT   WHAT CAN I DO? 51
- Strategies to Assist Memory 51
- The Big Three Risk Factors 52
- Foods to Eat 54
- Foods to Avoid 55
- Other Risk Factors to Work On 57
- Medications to Treat Alzheimer's Disease 66

CHAPTER NINE   HOW CAN I PREPARE FOR MY FUTURE? 69
- Knowledge is Power 69
- Long-Term Planning 70
- Decisions About Health 71
- Other Important Decisions 74

CONCLUSION 77

REFERENCES 79

Achieving Your Best Brain Health with Mild Cognitive Impairment

INTRODUCTION

Have you or a loved-one become increasingly concerned about your memory? Maybe you suspect that you are experiencing Mild Cognitive Impairment (MCI), or maybe someone such as your physician has suggested that you have MCI. Symptoms of cognitive change can bring with it feelings of anxiety, uncertainty, and the desire to learn more.

The purpose of this book is to help educate and guide you through a diagnosis of Mild Cognitive Impairment or early memory loss. It is meant to help answer many of your questions and empower you with knowledge to live your life to the fullest potential.

Kari Herman

CHAPTER ONE
Brain Basics

In order to understand why our brains are changing, we must first have a basic understanding of the brain. For the purposes of this book, this section will be kept to a somewhat simplified version.

Being the body's control center, the brain is undeniably an amazing organ. It is protected by the bony skull, and bathed and cushioned by cerebrospinal fluid. As adults, our brains weigh approximately 3 pounds. They are delicate and fragile powerhouses. Let's look at the different parts of the brain.

Cerebellum

The cerebellum is a small part of the back of the brain. The biggest responsibility of our cerebellum is our movement related functions, such as balance and coordination.

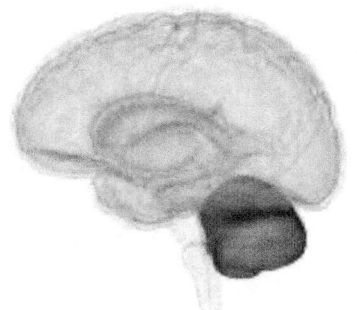
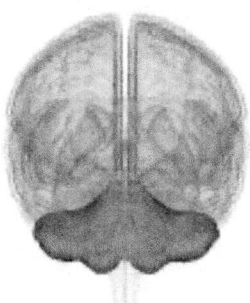

Brain Stem

The brain stem is an even smaller part of the brain that is found protected at the bottom. The brain stem is an extremely important part of our nervous system. It relays messages from the brain to the body. It is responsible for our most basic processes, such as controlling breathing, blood pressure, and other automatic functions such as consciousness and sleep cycles.

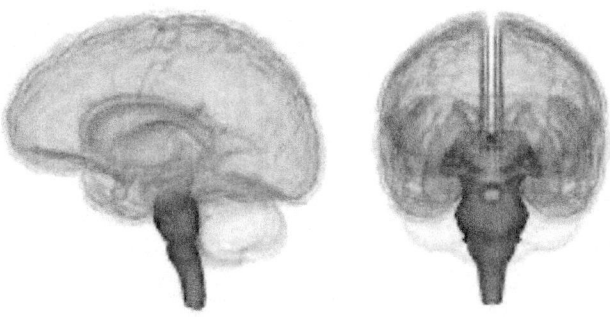

Cerebrum

The cerebrum is the largest part of our brain. It includes a right and a left side. Interestingly, the right side of our brain controls the left side of our body and vice versa. The cerebrum is where our thoughts, memories, and movements are housed. It has four lobes on each side of the brain that have been able to be mapped to tell us what areas of the brain are responsible for which processes.

Achieving Your Best Brain Health with Mild Cognitive Impairment

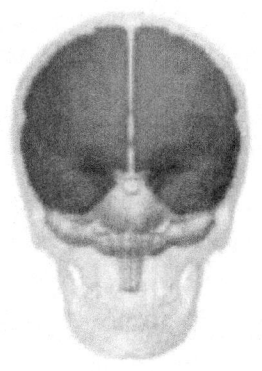

The Four Lobes of the Brain

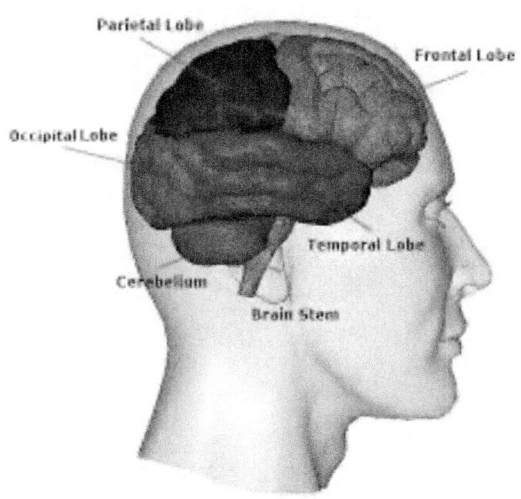

Kari Herman

The frontal lobes sit above the eyes and are the largest of the four lobes. They are responsible for the following functions:

- Personality, behavior, and emotions
- Judgement, planning, and problem solving
- Intelligence, concentration, and self-awareness
- Certain motor activities and speech

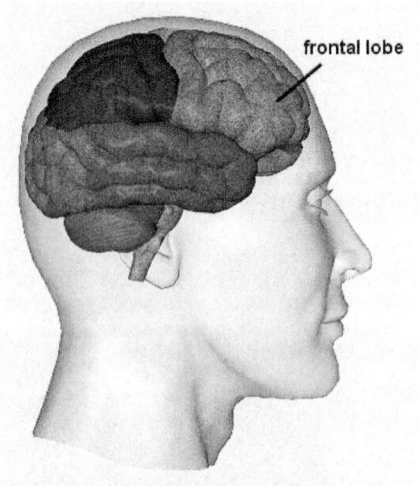

The parietal lobes are at the crown of the head and specialize in the following functions:

- Language
- The senses
- Visual and spatial perception

Achieving Your Best Brain Health with Mild Cognitive Impairment

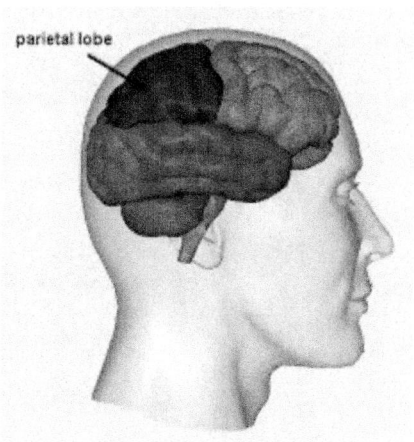

The occipital lobes are in the back of the brain. These areas specialize in interpreting vision.

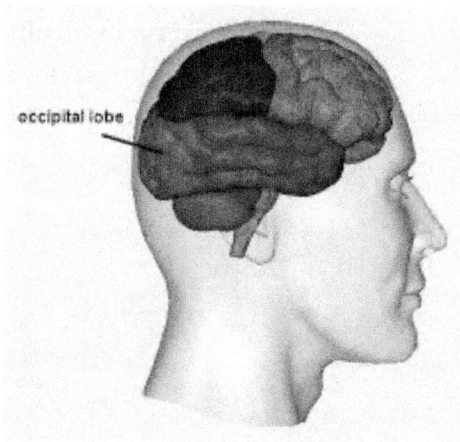

The temporal lobes are above the ears. These parts of the brain are responsible for processing sensory input (visual and

auditory), and for the formation of memories and memory storage which we will discuss further throughout the book.

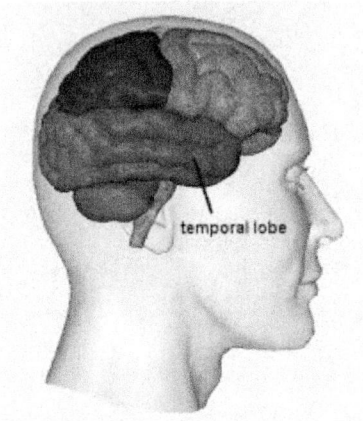

Cerebral Cortex

The cerebral cortex is the outermost layer or surface of the cerebrum. It has a folded appearance with "wiggly hills" (gyri) and "valleys" (sulci). The cerebral cortex is where approximately 86 billion nerve cells (neurons) are housed. This area is called our gray matter. It is the area of the brain where most information processing occurs.

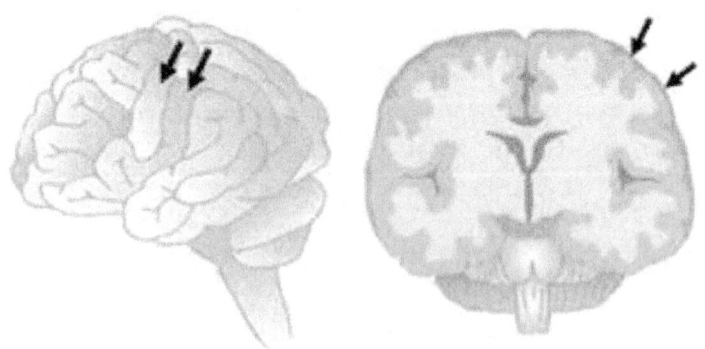

Achieving Your Best Brain Health with Mild Cognitive Impairment

The Hippocampi

The hippocampi are found in the inner folds of the temporal lobes. They are where memories are processed, indexed, and retrieved. The hippocampi are also where new short term memories are turned into long term memories. These long-term memories are then stored elsewhere in the brain. The hippocampi also help to regulate emotions.

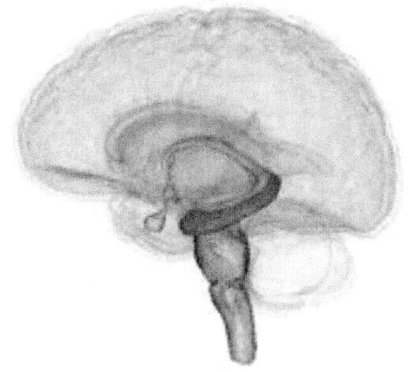 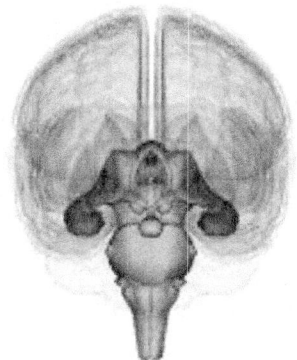

Neurons

Neurons are brain cells that are composed of a body, axon, and dendrites. The brain communicates and functions by sending chemical messengers called neurotransmitters from one neuron to the other. All sensations, movements, thoughts, memories, and feelings are the result of signals that pass through these neurons.

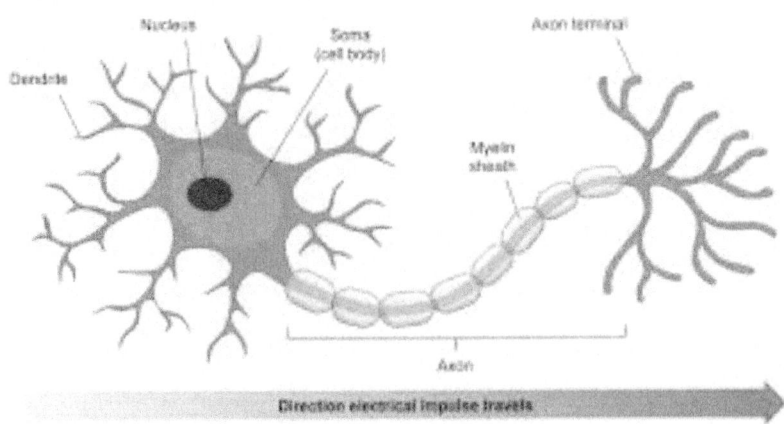

Blood Supply Network

The normal function of the brain's control centers is dependent upon an adequate supply of oxygen and nutrients through a dense network of blood vessels. Our brain receives 15-20% of our blood supply. Brain tissue that is deprived of oxygen and glucose as a result of compromised blood supply is likely to sustain damage and nerve cell death.

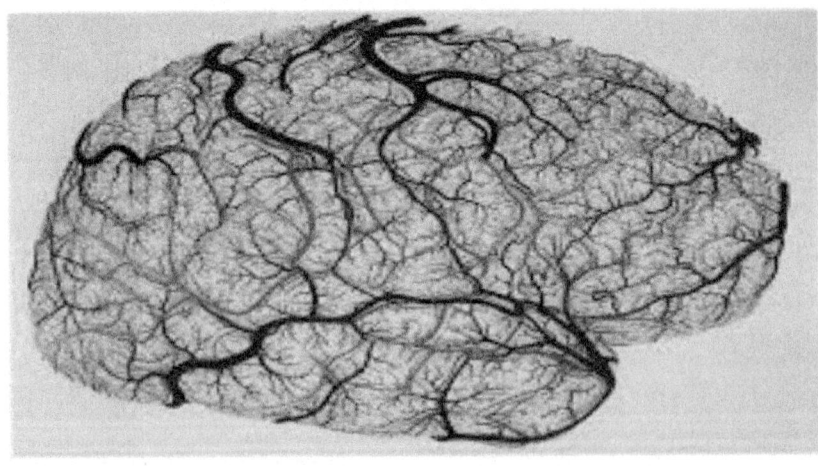

CHAPTER TWO
Memory Processing

Stages of Memory

Sensory memory lasts a few seconds or less, just long enough to respond to something you sense.

Short term memory is also a temporary memory. Here, new information is both stored and sorted before it is recorded permanently or lost through lack of attention. The capacity of short term memory is limited to 5-7 items. Items are held as long as you continue to give them your attention.

Working memory is the term for the processing of information you are holding in short term memory. Typically it is this processing of thoughts and feelings which moves experiences into your long term memory. Collecting new information, thinking about it, talking about it, and any other related action helps ensure that the information is retained and further integrated into long term memory.

Long term memory is our memory bank. The storage space is unlimited.

Memory Testing

According to the Alzheimer's Association, 82 percent of seniors agree that it is important to have their thinking and memory checked, but only 16 percent say they receive regular cognitive assessments.

MCI however cannot be diagnosed by neuropsychological tests alone, clinical judgement is always required.

Normal Age-Related Changes

As we get older, all of our body systems generally decline, including the brain. Aging causes changes in the size and blood flow to the brain, as well as other changes that affect our cognitive abilities. It has been found that **the brain becomes fully developed around the age of 22 and** the overall size of the brain starts to decrease in size around the age of 60-70. The areas most affected with aging occurs to the frontal lobes (the intellectual and higher thought process area) and the hippocampus (the memory center). The cerebral cortex becomes thinner and there are decreased neurotransmitter chemicals to allow neurons to communicate together as well.

Even though as many as 20 percent of 70 year olds perform just as well as 20 year olds on cognitive tests, there are many common cognitive changes that occur with normal aging. These changes can include:

- More effort required in learning something new and committing things to memory.

- Multi-tasking difficulties due to slower processing and planning of parallel tasks

Achieving Your Best Brain Health with Mild Cognitive Impairment

- Problems recalling names and appointments, but remembering them later
- Misplacing items, but being able to retrace your steps and find them
- Sometimes having trouble finding the right word

Everyone has memory lapses. We forget because we are human. Our many thoughts, feelings, needs, and desires are in frequent competition. Each of us live in the midst of a wide range of choices, stimulations to the senses, and demands of our attention. Sometimes this attention is grabbed away from one pressing concern by another with a louder voice. This often creates a memory lapse.

If you are experiencing memory loss, it does not necessarily mean that you have dementia. There are many circumstances including normal aging itself that can cause a person to have cognitive changes.

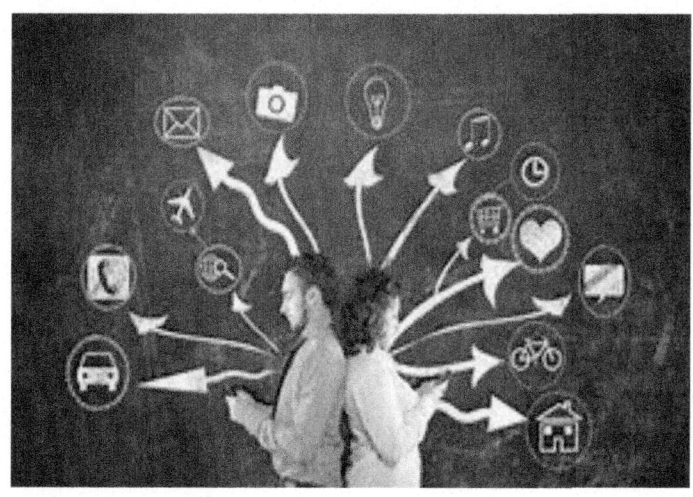

Reversible Causes of Memory Impairment

There are many possibly reversible medical issues that can cause memory or cognitive changes. Your physician will help to rule out these causes. Most of these reversible conditions are easily identified by a careful history, physical examination, brain imaging, and routine laboratory tests. Often these conditions can result in a return of normal cognitive abilities to your baseline, or improvement with treatment.

Some examples of potentially reversible cognitive problems include:

- Delirium (a fast-evolving condition resembling dementia) from metabolic issues:

    Dehydration
    Electrolyte imbalances
    Infections such as bladder infections, or respiratory infections

- Mismanaged medications or toxic reactions to medications

- Thyroid, parathyroid, or hormonal imbalances

- Vitamin deficiencies

- Nutritional deficiencies or anemia

- Cerebral hematomas (blood clot in the brain), TIA's (mini-strokes), or tumors

- Alcohol related

- Depression induced

Achieving Your Best Brain Health with Mild Cognitive Impairment

- Encephalopathy (swelling of the brain)
- Normal Pressure Hydrocephalous

Kari Herman

CHAPTER THREE
Mild Cognitive Impairment

Everyone experiences forgetfulness at times. This can include misplacing your keys or forgetting someone's name on occasion. Mild Cognitive Impairment is diagnosed as a cognitive state that falls somewhere between normal aging changes in the brain and mild dementia or Alzheimer's Disease. It has further been defined as a slight impairment in cognitive function, typically memory, with essentially otherwise normal performance. It is estimated that approximately 10-20% of adults over the age of 65 have MCI.

MCI becomes diagnosed when you or your loved-ones start to notice consistent or increasing changes that are slight, but not normal for people your age. Importantly, these changes are not serious enough to interfere with your daily life, activities, or independence. These changes occur in the mental functions of memory and thinking skills.

Some examples of the symptoms of MCI include the following:

- Forgetting important things such as appointment or engagements

- Difficulty staying on track during conversations, books, or movies

- Changes or difficulty with making decisions or understanding instructions

- Needing to concentrate harder for more complex tasks

- Losing things more often

- Word finding difficulties

- Changes with poor judgement beyond making a bad decision once in a while

- Problems with sense of smell

Types of MCI

MCI is categorized into two major types.

Amnestic MCI refers to changes and challenges specifically with memory, such as forgetting recent information or details of conversation for example.

Non-amnestic MCI is a second category of Mild Cognitive Impairment that involves changes in areas other than memory, such as attention and concentration, executive function, language and visual skills.

Some people have deficits in only one of these areas or have small deficits in multiple areas of cognition. Everyone is different.

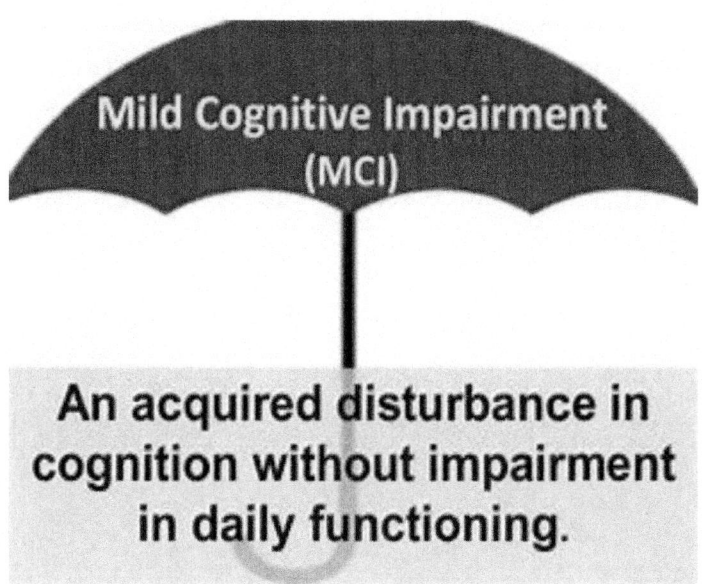

Possible Causes of MCI

Research is showing that MCI is often the result of some of the changes that happen in the brain for people experiencing dementia or Alzheimer's Disease. Changes in the brain found upon autopsy of those experiencing MCI have included:

1. The presence of plaques. Plaques are abnormal clusters of protein fragments called beta amyloid, that build up between nerve cells. These plaques form around dead brain cells. As they form, they stick together in clumps which prevents neurons from communicating to each other.

2. Dead and dying nerve cells contain neurofibrillary tangles, which are made up of twisted strands of a different protein called Tau. The Tau proteins bunch together and twist around each other. The tangles twist up parallel nerve cell fibers, causing them to fall apart, disintegrate, and destroy the neurons vital transport system within and eventually destroy the neuron.

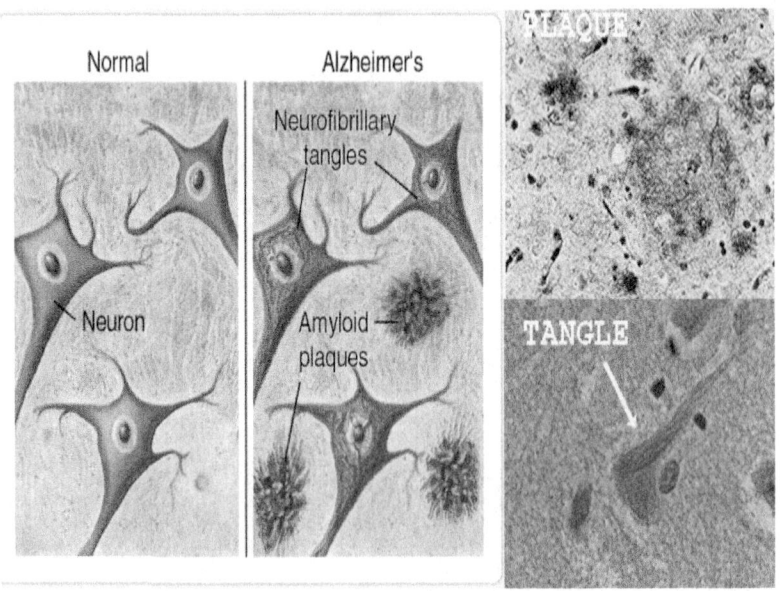

3. Lewy bodies are abnormal aggregates of a protein called alpha-synuclein that develop in nerve cells and disrupt the brain's normal functioning. These clumps form inside neurons throughout the brain. This causes neurons to become damaged and die. These deposits affect chemical messengers in the brain also.

Achieving Your Best Brain Health with Mild Cognitive Impairment

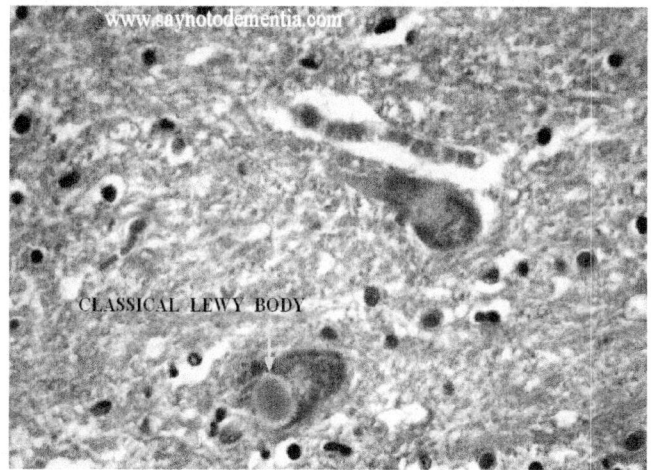

4. Small strokes, microvascular changes, or impaired blood flow problems can damage and eventually kill cells anywhere in the body. Because the brain is so rich in blood vessels it is particularly vulnerable.

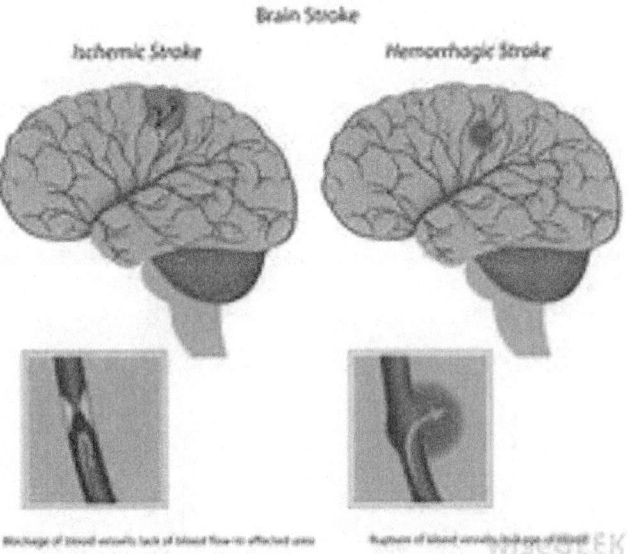

5. Brain imaging studies of people with MCI have also found shrinking of the hippocampus. This is present in people with Alzheimer's Disease as well and is where memories are consolidated from short term memory to long term memory.

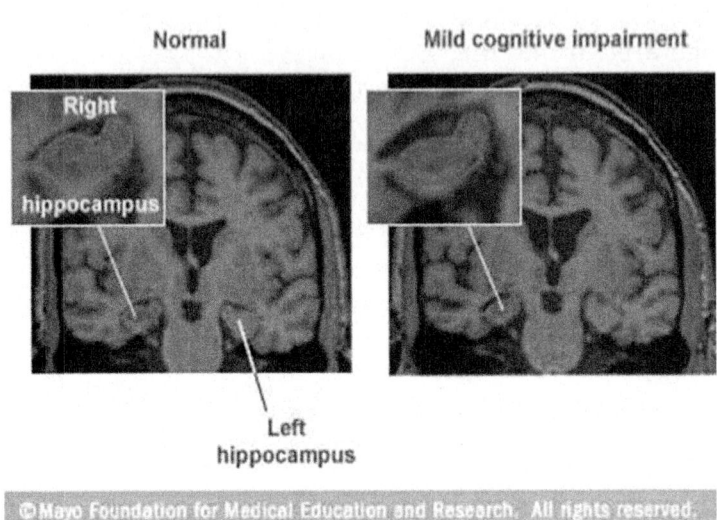

Achieving Your Best Brain Health with Mild Cognitive Impairment

6. Ventricle enlargement is also seen with MCI, and is caused by shrinking of brain tissue. The ventricles of the brain are a communicating network of cavities that produce cerebrospinal fluid and allow it to flow around and cushion the brain and spinal cord.

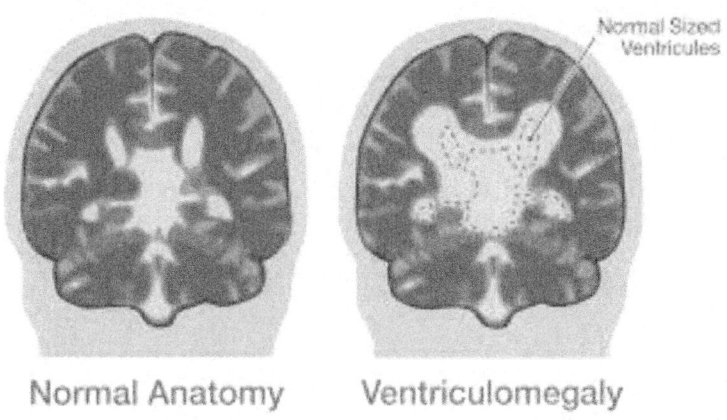

Normal Anatomy   Ventriculomegaly

7. Decreased levels of glucose use is another change in the brain suspected of causing memory changes seen with MCI. The key role of glucose in the body is fuel for energy, and the brain depends completely on glucose to operate normally. Brain functions such as thinking, learning and memory are closely tied to glucose levels and how effectively the brain utilizes glucose.

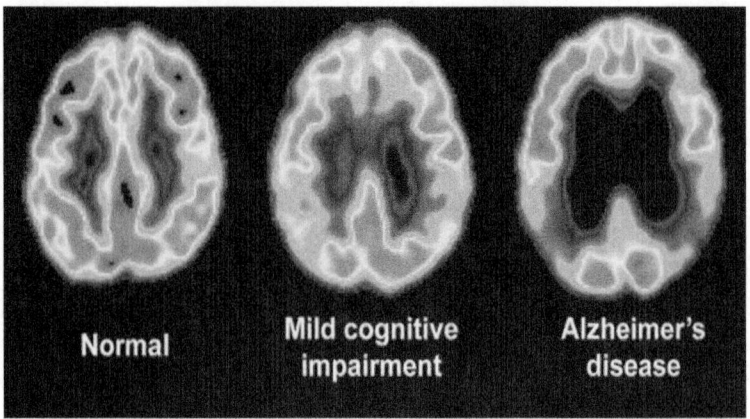

8. Other risk factors for mild cognitive impairment include:

- Increasing age

- Having the gene APOE4. A genetic allele found in 10–20 percent of the population.

- And many other risk factors such as smoking, diabetes, hypertension, increased cholesterol, lack of physical exercise, and other risk factors that will be discussed later in the book.

Prognosis

Some people living with MCI will never get worse, a few will improve, and some will go on to develop a progressive dementia or Alzheimer's disease.

It is not possible to determine a specific person's outcome. Studies suggest that approximately 10–15 percent of those with

Achieving Your Best Brain Health with Mild Cognitive Impairment

MCI will go on to develop dementia each year after diagnosis. Within 4 years, approximately 50 percent of those with MCI will experience a progression to dementia. People with amnestic MCI are more likely to develop Alzheimer's disease than those with non-amnestic MCI.

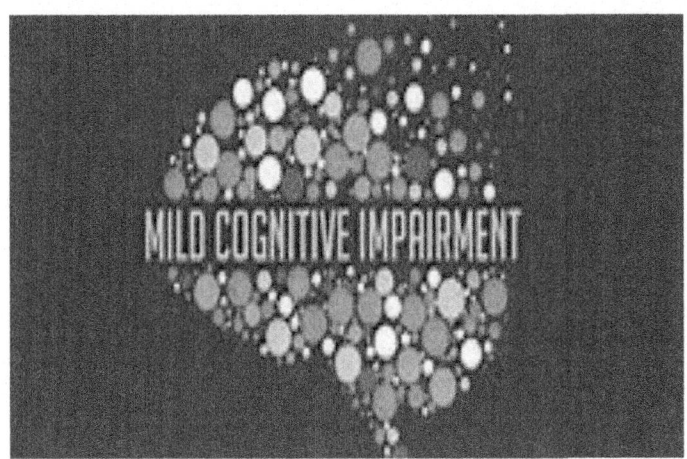

Kari Herman

CHAPTER FOUR
MCI and Mild Dementia Caused by Alzheimer's Disease

In the early stage of Alzheimer's disease, a person may function independently. He or she may still drive, work, and be part of social activities. Despite this, the person may feel as if he or she is having memory lapses, such as forgetting familiar words or the location of everyday objects. The symptoms of dementia are more severe than simple forgetfulness and involve learning, thinking, reasoning, and communicating. The symptoms soon start to impact work, social activities, and family life. Friends, family, and others close to the individual begin to notice difficulties. During a detailed medical interview, doctors may be able to detect problems in memory or concentration. Common difficulties of Dementia include:

- Short term memory impairment & confusion

- Problems coming up with the right word or name for an item

- Trouble remembering names when introduced to new people

- Challenges performing tasks in social or work settings

- Forgetting material that was just read

- Losing or misplacing valuable objects

- Increased trouble with planning and organizing

Alzheimer's disease typically progresses slowly in three stages – mild (early stage), moderate (middle stage), and severe (late stage). Since this disease affects people in different ways, the timing and severity of symptoms varies from person to person through the stages differently. The symptoms progressively and slowly worsen over time. On average, a person with Alzheimer's lives approximately 8 years after diagnosis, however this range can be 4-20 years.

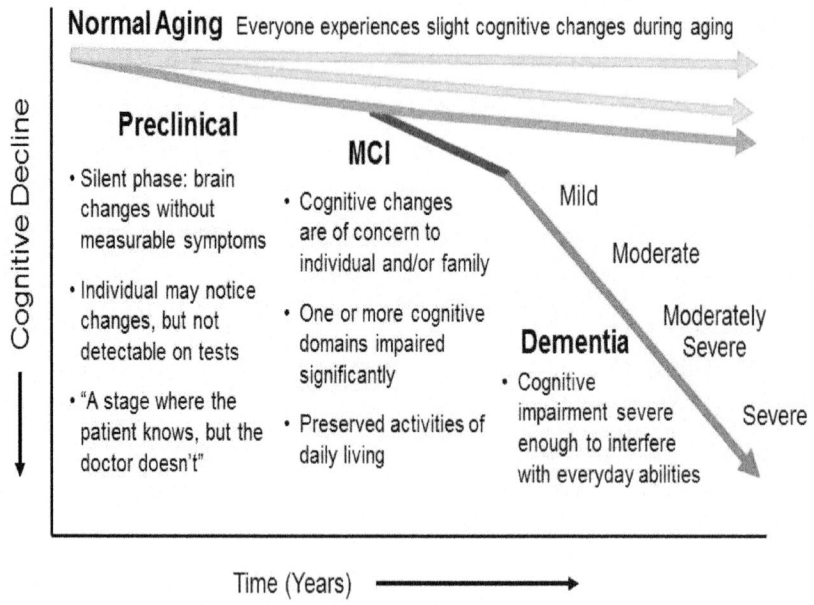

Achieving Your Best Brain Health with Mild Cognitive Impairment

There are over 100 conditions that cause memory impairment. At least 84 of those conditions cause a progressive dementia. Alzheimer's is the most common form of progressive dementia. It accounts for 60-80 percent of all dementia cases. The other most frequent form of dementia include:

- Vascular dementia
- Lewy body dementia
- Frontotemporal dementia

We will look further into these types of dementia for comparison.

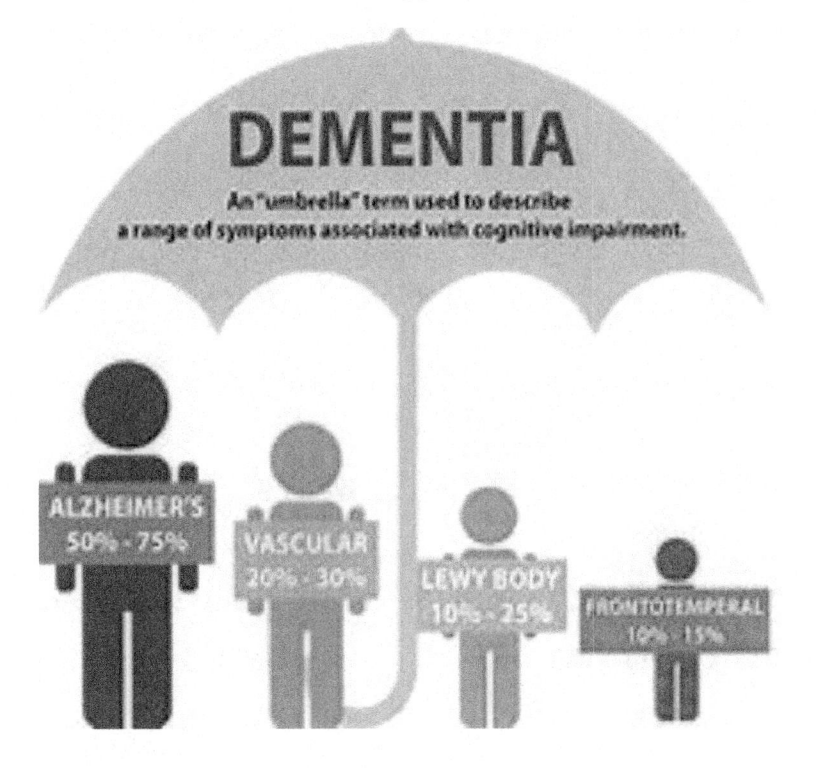

DEMENTIA
An "umbrella" term used to describe a range of symptoms associated with cognitive impairment.

ALZHEIMER'S 50% - 75%
VASCULAR 20% - 30%
LEWY BODY 10% - 25%
FRONTOTEMPORAL 10% - 15%

Vascular Dementia

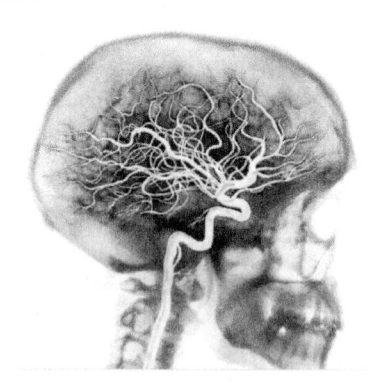

Vascular dementia used to be called "Multi-Infarct" or "Post-Stroke Dementia". It is considered the second most common type of dementia. Vascular dementia (VD) is caused by brain cell damage from microscopic bleeding, larger incidents of stroke, and/or blood vessel blockage.

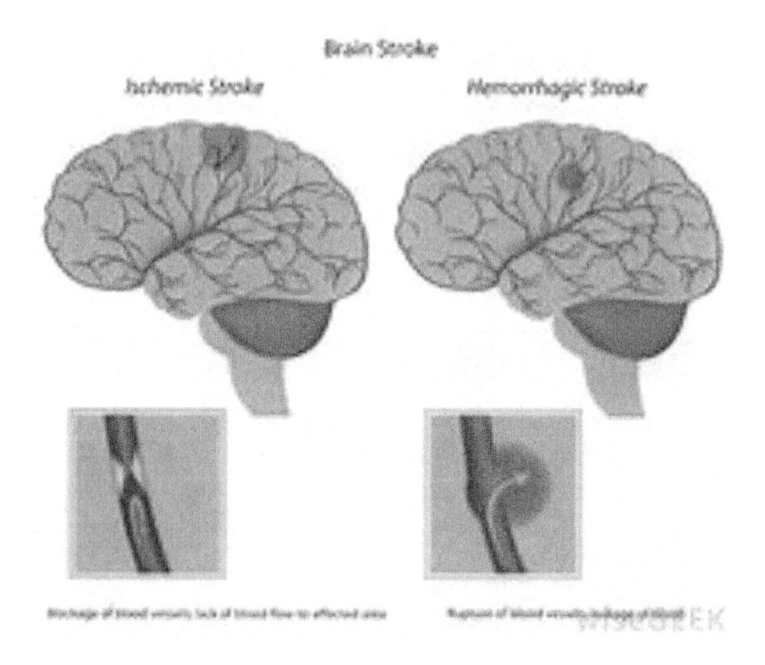

Achieving Your Best Brain Health with Mild Cognitive Impairment

The symptoms of Vascular dementia often begin suddenly, frequently after a stroke. Early symptoms of this disease depends on the area of the brain affected. This often includes issues such as impaired judgement or the ability to make plans, as opposed to memory loss. The following symptoms also occur more commonly in Vascular dementia, as opposed to Alzheimer's disease. Each person is unique however.

- Unsteady gait
- One-sided neglect or weakness
- Incontinence
- Mood and behavioral changes
- Wandering

Vascular dementia also has a telling "stair-step decline". There will be sudden changes in abilities, as opposed to a slow, steady decline as is the case with Alzheimer's. The life expectancy of someone experiencing VD is highly variable and often depends on improvement of any risk factors that contributed to the vascular issues such as:

- High blood pressure
- Diabetes
- Smoking
- High cholesterol
- Atrial fibrillation

For these reasons, Vascular dementia is referred to as one of the most preventable forms of dementia. It is also important to know that VD and Alzheimer's disease often occur together. This is called a "mixed dementia."

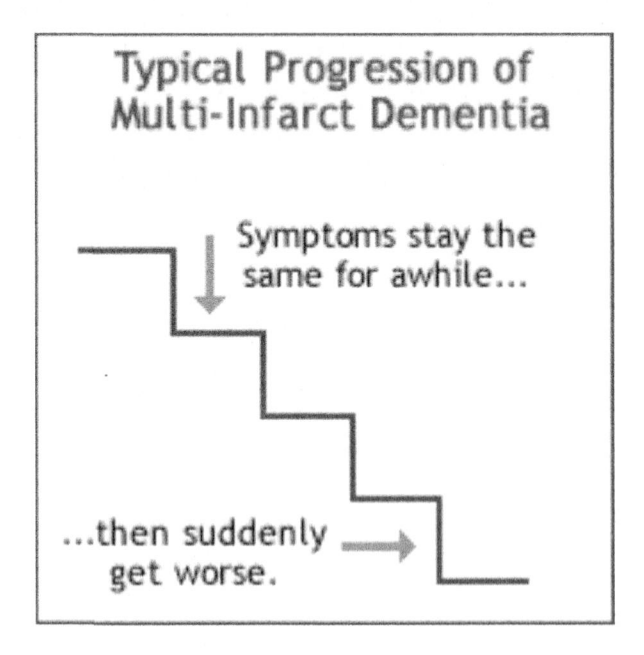

Typical Progression of Multi-Infarct Dementia

Symptoms stay the same for awhile... then suddenly get worse.

Lewy Body Dementia

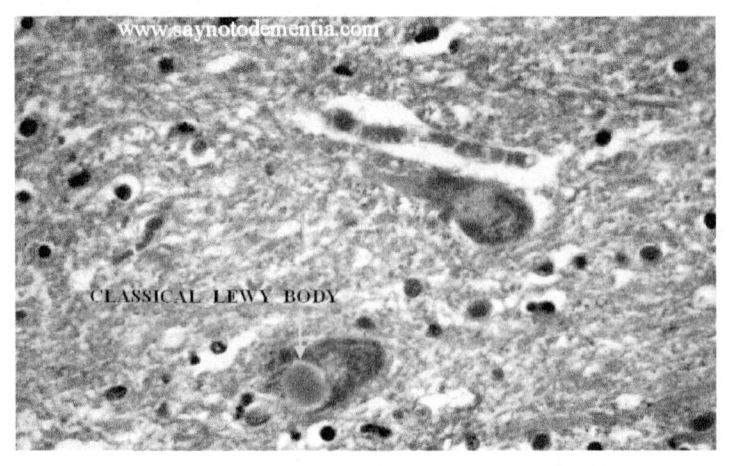

CLASSICAL LEWY BODY

Achieving Your Best Brain Health with Mild Cognitive Impairment

Lewy body dementia (LBD) competes with Vascular dementia as the second most common type of dementia. It occurs sporadically, in people with no known family history. Generally the most common age of onset is 50-85 years of age. Lewy Body Dementia is caused by the build up of Lewy Bodies (clumps of alpha-synuclein protein) in the brain. It often occurs as a "mixed dementia" along with Alzheimer's disease or Vascular Dementia. Lewy Body Dementia and Parkinson's Disease Dementia start out differently, however have similar symptoms as progression happens.

Progressive cognitive decline is the central feature of this disease combined with additional defining features including:

- Pronounced fluctuations in alertness and attention
- Recurrent, well-formed, visual hallucinations early in the disease
- Visuospatial difficulties
- Parkinson's like symptoms and falls
- REM sleep disorder
- Autonomic nervous system problems (such as blood pressure, dizziness, and incontinence for example)

Frontotemporal Dementia

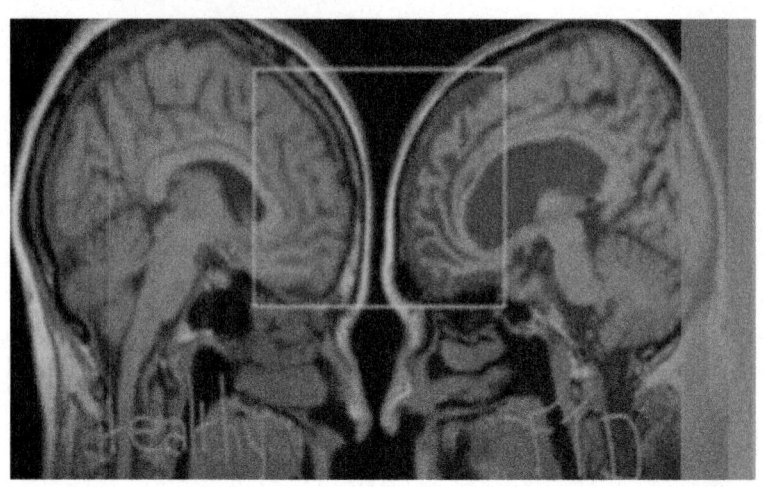

Frontotemporal dementia (FTD) symptoms usually appear when a person is 45-65 years of age. Experts believe that FTD accounts for approximately 10-20 percent of all progressive dementias. It affects the frontal lobes and the temporal lobes. Many people with Frontotemporal Dementia have a family history of dementia.

The first, defining symptoms include changes in personality, behavior, and/or language. Memory loss occurs later in the disease. There are often problems with maintaining normal interactions and following social expectations. Specific examples can include

- Impolite or socially inappropriate behaviors
- Compulsive or repetitive behaviors
- Increased appetite
- Movement and language problems

Achieving Your Best Brain Health with Mild Cognitive Impairment

Frontotemporal dementia is an umbrella term for a group of brain disorders including:

- Behavioral Variant FTD
- Pick's Disease
- Primary Progressive Aphasia
- Semantic Dementia
- Corticobasal Degeneration
- FTD – Motor Neuron Disease
- Progressive Supranuclear Palsy

Additional Types of Dementia include:

- Parkinson's Disease Dementia
- Huntington's Disease
- Chronic Traumatic Encephalopathy
- Wernicke-Korsakoff Syndrome
- Creutzfeldt-Jakob Disease
- HIV Associated Dementia
- And many more

Kari Herman

CHAPTER FIVE
Why I Should Pay Attention

Benefits of an Early Diagnosis

There are many benefits to being honest and proactive about the memory changes that you are noticing. Some people affected will chose to ignore or hide what is happening. This can lead to decreased coping, decreased cognition, and also can cause future challenges with families and loved ones. Some of the benefits of receiving an early diagnosis include the following:

- The ability to rule out and treat possible reversible conditions

- To provide an answer and validation for what is happening and the opportunity to gain knowledge

- A better ability to come up with a correct diagnosis

- To allow a better chance at benefitting from treatments such as risk factor management

- To allow time to develop crucial relationships with physicians and care providers

- The time, knowledge, and power to make your own life decisions for the future

- Earlier access to peer, support groups, and even research trials if interested

Working with Your Doctor

Sometimes getting an accurate diagnosis of MCI is difficult. Some reasons for this can include:

- Not all doctors are comfortable making these diagnoses because there is not a single, accurate test

- Some doctors feel inadequate in treating symptoms of these disorders

- Medications for treating dementias are fairly new and some doctors may not be familiar with or believe in their potential benefits

- It is possible for some people to sustain severe memory loss and still appear superficially "normal" to others, including their physicians for many years

- Dealing with a diagnosis of dementia often includes many complex psychosocial family matters that some doctors do not have adequate time to explore

- Many health insurances do not adequately reimburse physicians for their time and effort to deal with these disorders effectively

How well you and your doctor or care provider talk to each other is one of the most important parts of getting good health care. Talking with your doctor isn't always an easy thing to do, it takes time and effort on your part as well as the doctor's.

Achieving Your Best Brain Health with Mild Cognitive Impairment

Getting Ready for a Doctor's Appointment

- Make a list of your concerns and prioritize them

- Take your medication bottles with you

- Make sure you can see and hear as well as possible

- Consider bringing a family member or friend

- Be sure to update your doctor on things that have happened since your last visit

- If you are tech savy, sign up for online health services

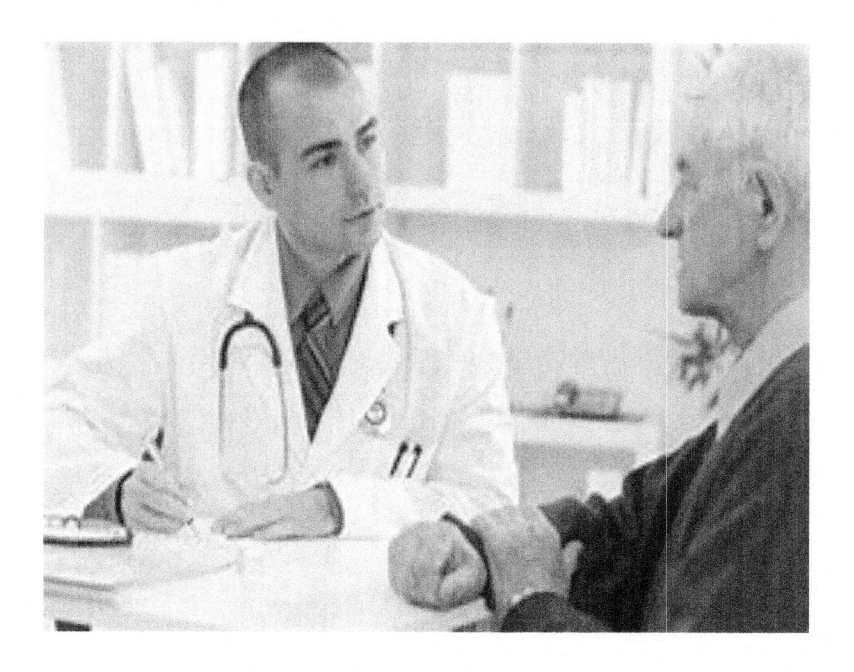

How a Diagnosis is Made

The first and most important step to getting a diagnosis is self-identification. When this doesn't happen, many people go without a diagnosis. This can result in the ability to cope, and attempts at pushing back at progression being unrealized.

After self-identification, the next step is to see your primary care provider. This is hopefully a provider who is familiar with you who will be able to assess changes from your previous baseline status. You can expect the following from your provider:

- A complete history and physical exam
- Assessment of changes in function
- Possible request for input from a loved one
- Blood work
- Memory screening
- Ruling out of possible reversible cognitive changes
- Possible brain imaging
- Possible referrals to specialists

Specialists

Neuropsychologist: A psychologist who has completed special training in testing memory and in diagnosing and treating these illnesses

Achieving Your Best Brain Health with Mild Cognitive Impairment

Geriatric Specialist: A physician who has specialized postgraduate education and experience in the medical care of older adults

Neurologist: A physician who specializes in disorders of the brain and central nervous system

Several biomarkers for Alzheimer's Disease have emerged in the last few years. However, even those these markers are present, there are not always symptoms of disease. These biomarkers include:

- Amyloid and Tau proteins in cerebrospinal fluid

- Hippocampal atrophy on an MRI

- Decreased glucose metabolism and amyloid presence as seen with a PET scan

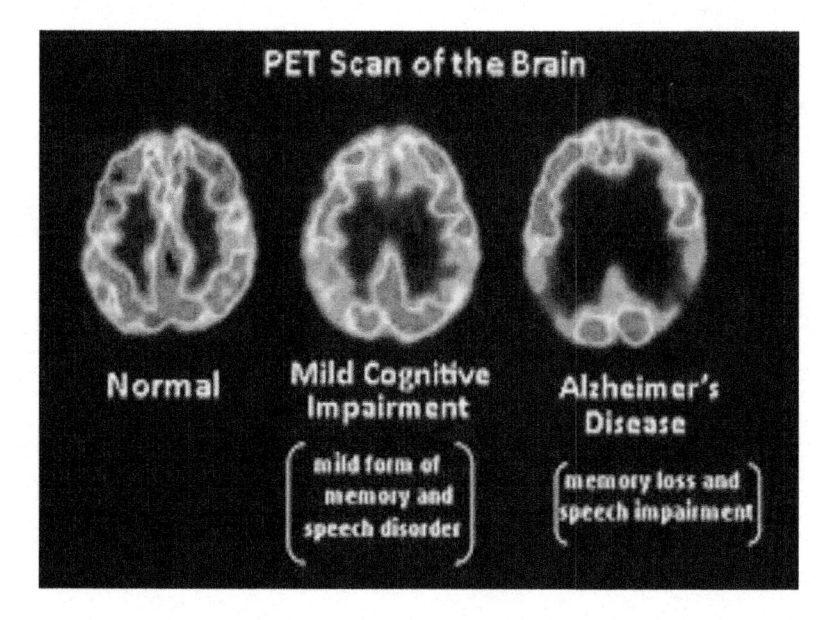

PET Scan of the Brain

Normal | Mild Cognitive Impairment (mild form of memory and speech disorder) | Alzheimer's Disease (memory loss and speech impairment)

Kari Herman

CHAPTER SIX
How Will I Go On?

Adjusting to a New Diagnosis

Although adjusting to a new diagnosis can be very difficult, it is important to know that there are several things you can do to experience and cope with this new journey. Each person will deal with their symptoms differently.

Paying attention to and acknowledging your emotions is important. Understand that experiencing a wide range of emotions is completely normal. Possible emotions and feelings can include:

- Shock and disbelief

- Denial

- Anger

- Grief and depression

- Fear

- Relief

You may experience all or some of these emotions. There is no specific expected order of emotions. You may move back and forth amongst them. The goal is to be able to experience some level of acceptance of your MCI diagnosis. Acknowledging it will help you be able to focus on ways to live your life to the fullest.

One research study found that almost one half of participants diagnosed with MCI or early dementia found positive aspects of receiving a formal diagnosis. This includes feelings of:

- Validation

- Appreciation and acceptance of life

- Less concern about failure

- Self-reflection, tolerance of others, and courage to face problems in life

- Strengthened relationships and new opportunities to meet people

Coping

You probably have many questions and concerns. The best thing you can do is to educate yourself and to set up a support system. Other things that you can do to cope include:

- Learn as much as you can. Knowledge is power

- If you are sad or angry, allow yourself to cry

- Scream or punch into a pillow if you need to

- Share your diagnosis with close friends and family who can help

- Keep connected with family and friends for social support

Achieving Your Best Brain Health with Mild Cognitive Impairment

- Consider joining a support group. It will help to talk to others going through the same or similar experiences

- Document your personal journey to reflect and help put things into perspective in a journal

- Reach out for holistic and spiritual care

- Become an advocate. Research, promote, advocate for MCI

- Be patient with yourself and ask family to as well

- Slow down and prioritize your tasks

- Exercise, or use arts or music to release emotions

- Focus on your abilities and not limitations

- Remember you are much more than simply someone with MCI

- Live an active and productive life

- Live one day at a time

- Use positive self talk, "easy does it", "first things first", or "how important is it?"

- Start a gratitude list

- Avoid destructive behaviors such as drugs, alcohol, overeating, or outbursts of anger

Kari Herman

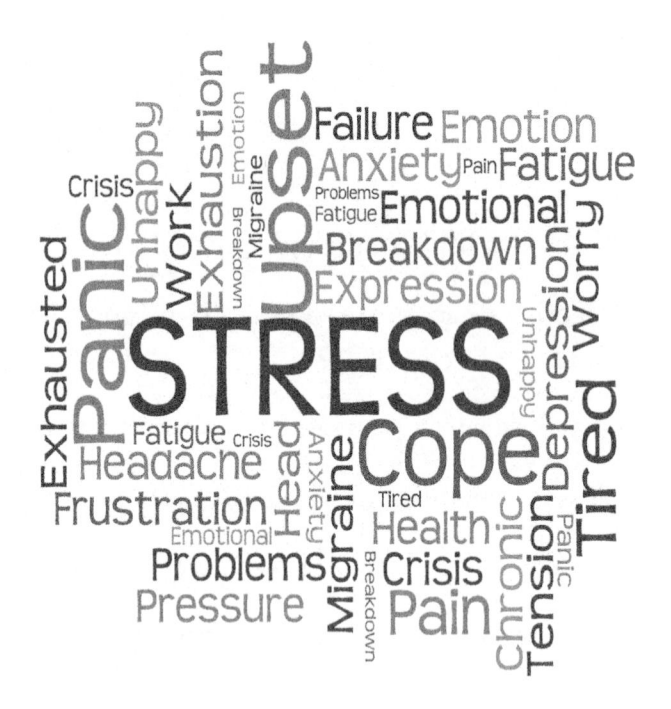

CHAPTER SEVEN
How Will the Roles in my Life Change?

Changes

Memory changes may affect your relationships. While your abilities may change over time, it is important to understand that you have the ability to live well in your relationships. This may depend on how you choose to continue to be a partner in your relationships. You may feel as if you are going to lose those things that give you a sense of who you are, for example your job, the things you love to do, your accomplishments, or your role as a partner. These represent only parts of who you actually are. Remember, your personal sense of self comes from within you.

It is imperative to remember that you are still the same person that you were before your memory changes started to occur. Although it may take time for some friends and family to adjust to your changes, it is also very important that you not withdraw from friends and family. Withdrawal can have many negative consequences on not only your brain health, but also your quality of life.

It is important to identify the roles in your life that are the most important to you, to allow you to focus on them. Consider what roles you currently have whether it be in your career, with your family, with friends, or with your church for example. Is it time to retire, due to the extra effort required to perform your job and the desire to focus on other roles and responsibilities?

Kari Herman

Marital relationships may change when one person is living with memory changes. The person living with MCI may lose confidence and need more support from their loved one. The care partner may likely have fears and frustrations also. This can lead to stress for both the person living with the changes, and the person supporting them.

However, some people living with MCI experience strengthened relationships.

Some suggestions to keep your relationships positive and productive include:

- Be open about your feelings and share them

- Be specific about how you would like to continue relationships and how you would like to be treated.

- Learn to ask for help. Tell others how they can help.

- Strengthen trusting relationships. Focus on those relationships which are supportive, and show your gratitude for the people you love and appreciate

- Reevaluate relationships. Consider letting go of some people who are unable to support you or unable to have a positive presence in your life

- See yourself as unique and human. You have much left to offer and experience!

Achieving Your Best Brain Health with Mild Cognitive Impairment

Caregiver Wellness

> "The capacity to care is the main thing which gives life its deepest meaning and significance." Pablo Casals

Care partners are loved ones that can be friends or family. Someone who is close and supportive to you. It is important to remember that our care partners can experience stress as they watch you change and maybe even struggle at times.

Care partners must care for themselves as well to maintain a healthy relationship with someone experiencing memory changes. It has been found that caregivers die at a rate of 63 percent higher than people the same age who are not caring for someone with memory loss. For this reason, caregivers should maintain a sense of a separate identity alone along with their role of caregiver. Most of the suggested ideas for coping in Chapter 3 are very applicable for care partners as well.

It is also helpful to accept changes as they occur and just do the best you can. People with cognitive changes often change over time and so do their needs. Accept that changes are part of the process and journey.

Kari Herman

Achieving Your Best Brain Health with Mild Cognitive Impairment

CHAPTER EIGHT
What Can I Do?

Strategies to Assist Memory

- Make sure to use a calendar
- Keep a notepad handy
- Outline a schedule for the day
- Keep routines
- Consider using an automatic dispensing pill box
- Use bulletin boards
- Make use of technology reminders
- Organize important objects together (keys, money)
- Use clocks and watches that have dates
- Keep up to date with current news
- Use mnemonics and chunking
- Place mental aides in the bathrooms, bedrooms, and kitchens
- Leave voice messages for yourself
- Ask for support from family members

The Big Three Risk Factors

There is growing evidence that people can take steps to reduce their risk of dementia, push back at memory changes, and improve their overall brain health.

Blood Pressure: Recent research presented in the January 2019 Journal of the American Medical Association has found that high blood pressure causes damage to the blood vessels of the brain and that people with MCI tend to have this type of damage. High blood pressure can worsen these cognitive problems and result in changes. The study noted that intensive lowering of systolic blood pressure may prevent MCI, and possibly decrease the prevention of MCI to dementia. The American Heart Association currently recommends that blood pressure levels be below 120/80mmHg. This, however, must be individualized with your physician.

Besides having regular blood pressure checks and ensuring a healthy blood pressure, doing other healthy things that we will talk more about, will positively affect your blood pressure. This includes things such as exercise, a low sodium diet, and weight management for example

Exercise: Research suggests that mild-to-moderate physical activity may help delay or slow a decline in thinking skills, reduce stress, possibly help improve symptoms of depression, and may even reduce the risk of falls. Exercise also directly benefits brain cells by increasing blood and oxygen flow.

The recommended amount of healthy exercise is 150 minutes per week of moderate-intensity or 75 minutes of vigorous-intensity aerobic exercise. Research has found that any activity is better

Achieving Your Best Brain Health with Mild Cognitive Impairment

than none. One study by Spartano found that people who achieved 10,000 steps per day had larger brain volumes than those that got less than 5,000.

This exercise should be spread out over the week. Even short, 10 minute segments count. It is also recommended to do strengthening activities twice weekly doing weights, resistance bands, sit ups, or push-ups for example.

Check with your doctor about how much and what type of exercise is best and safe for you. If you have been inactive, work with your doctor and start slowly. Remember that getting some physical activity is better than getting none.

Diet: The best current evidence suggests that heart-healthy eating patterns, may help protect the brain. There are many differing opinions about which diet may be the best for brain health. Most commonly cited are the Mediterranean diet, The DASH diet, and the MIND diet. The MIND diet specifically zeroes in on foods in the Mediterranean and the DASH diets that have a positive effect on brain health.

The MIND diet stands for Mediterranean-DASH Intervention for Neurodegenerative Delay. It was developed by researchers at Rush University Medical Center in Chicago and has been shown to reduce the risk of developing Alzheimer's Disease by as much as 53 percent. The study reports that even those who followed this diet only moderately well reduced their risk by about a third. This diet is also believed to help slow the rate of cognitive decline and reduce the risk of MCI progressing to Alzheimer's Disease. It has been found that following this diet consistently over the years will provide you with the best brain protection. This diet breaks down recommendations into 10 "brain healthy food groups" a person should eat more of, and 5 "unhealthy food groups" to avoid.

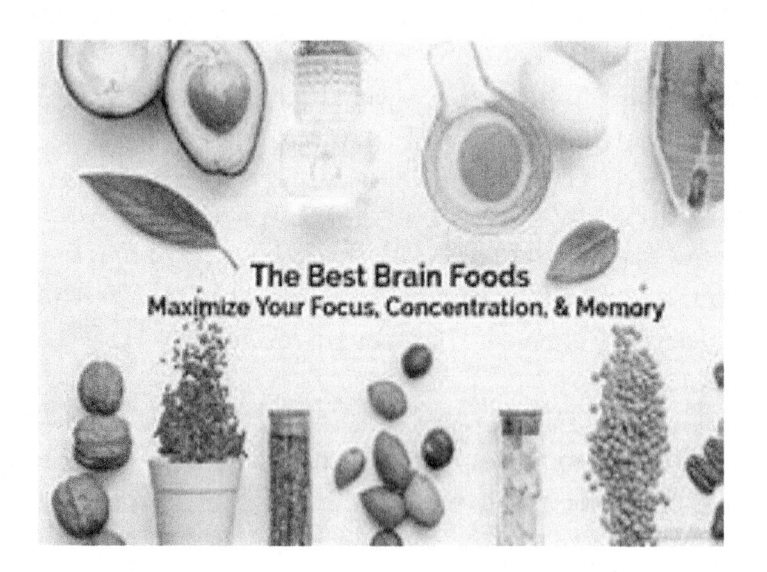

The Best Brain Foods
Maximize Your Focus, Concentration, & Memory

Foods to Eat

Leafy Green Vegetables such as kale, spinach, broccoli, collards, and other greens. At least 2 servings a week can help, but six or more servings per week provide the greatest brain benefits.

Other vegetables such as a salad or another type of vegetable every day is said to help.

Nuts make for a good and beneficial snack. They contain healthy fats, fiber, and antioxidants. Studies also show that they can help lower bad cholesterol as well. The recommendation is 5 servings per week.

Berries are the only fruit that are specifically recommended with the MIND diet, especially blueberries. Eating berries is encouraged at least twice weekly.

Beans are high in fiber and protein, low in calories and fat and are said to keep your mind sharp. Researchers recommend eating beans three times per week.

Whole grains are a key component of the MIND diet. At least three servings per day are recommended.

Fish is found to help protect brain function. The MIND diet recommends eating fish at least once per week.

Poultry is another part of brain-healthy eating with a recommendation for two or more servings per week.

Olive oil used as a primary cooking oil instead of other oils or fats is found to have greater protection against cognitive decline.

One drink of wine (or other "spirits") is recommended daily, especially red wine. Just one serving though.

Foods to Avoid

Red meat should be limited to no more than four servings per week to help protect brain health.

Butter and stick margarine should be limited to less than one tablespoon per day. Olive oil can often be used instead.

Cheese has been found to not be brain healthy. It is limited to no more than once per week.

Pastries and sweets can have a negative effect on brain health. The MIND diet recommends limiting yourself to no more than five of these a week.

Fried foods and fast foods are limited to no more than once per week for optimal brain health.

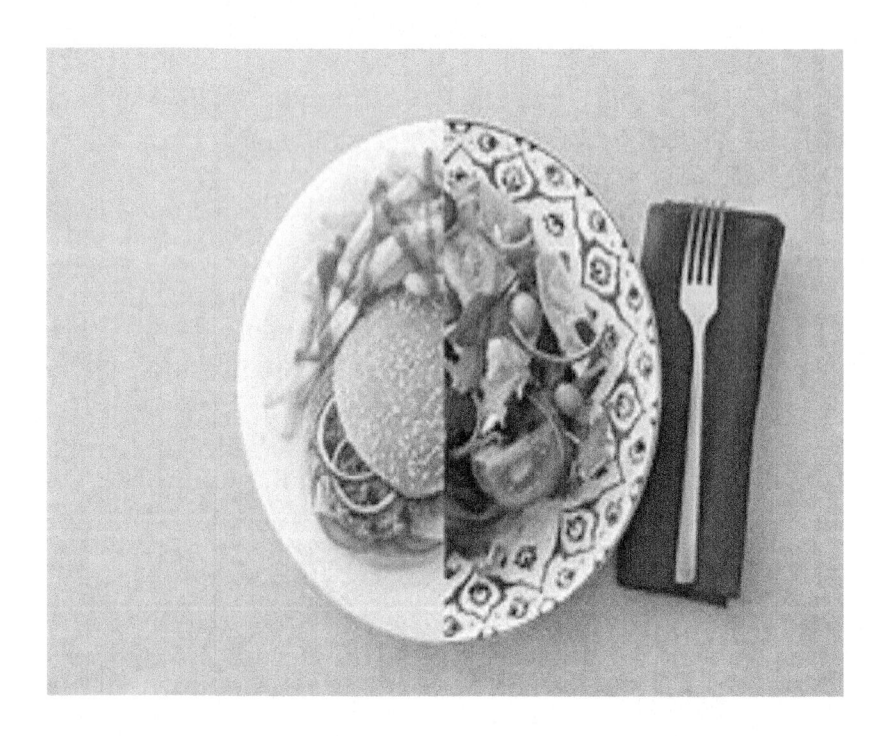

Achieving Your Best Brain Health with Mild Cognitive Impairment

Other Risk Factors to Work On

Depression: While it can be normal to feel sad about the changes you are experiencing, signs of depression are more severe and need to be treated.

Symptoms of depression can cause cognitive abilities to slow. Depression can be common in people living with MCI. Treatment can improve cognitive function and can also improve quality of life for those with MCI.

Some signs of depression can include:

- Feeling sad or hopeless most of the day, nearly every day
- Decreased interest in normally pleasurable activities
- Severe fatigue or loss of energy
- Difficulty concentrating, or making decisions
- Feelings of guilt or worthlessness
- Changes in appetite or sleeping patterns

If you are concerned you may have depression, please reach out to a care provider for evaluation and treatment.

There is no "one size fits all" treatment for depression. Some tips for treatment involve:

- Not relying on medications alone
- Get social support

- Realize that it takes time and patience

- Psychotherapy (talk treatment) can be extremely effective

- Medications may help relieve some of the symptoms of moderate to severe depression

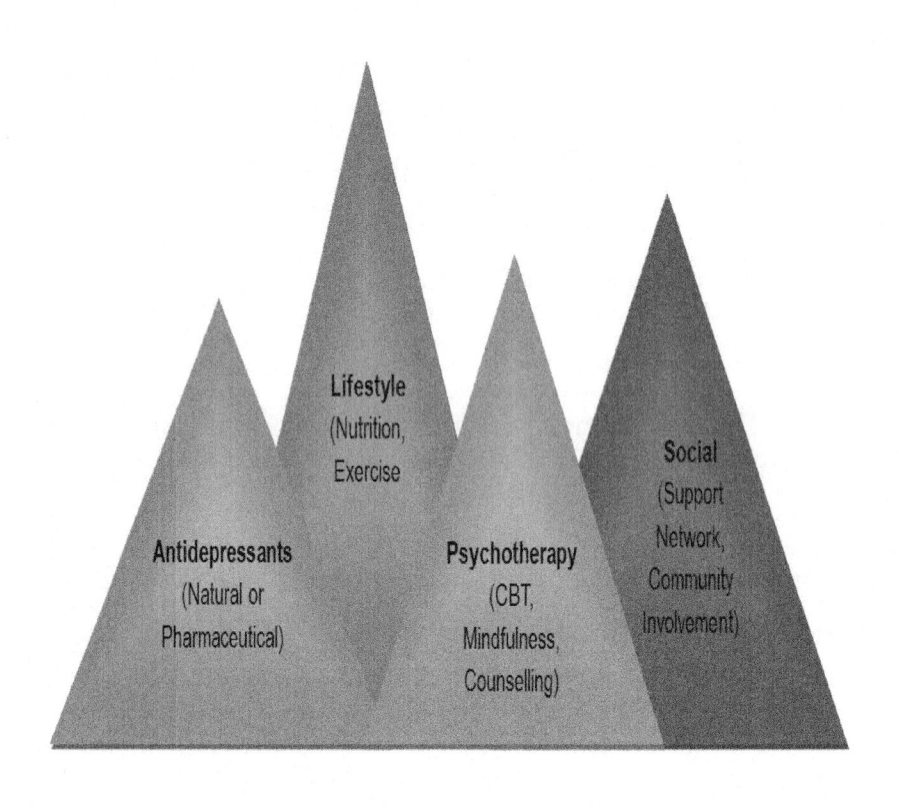

Antidepressants
(Natural or Pharmaceutical)

Lifestyle
(Nutrition, Exercise)

Psychotherapy
(CBT, Mindfulness, Counselling)

Social
(Support Network, Community Involvement)

Achieving Your Best Brain Health with Mild Cognitive Impairment

Non-Drug Approaches to Depression:

Exercise can help relieve depressive symptoms, by altering the mood-regulating chemicals norepinephrine and serotonin as well as by releasing endorphins. Any amount of exercise is better than none and it is especially helpful to do in the am.

Maintaining a predictable daily routine is very helpful to utilize the best times of the day, prioritize, and prevent fatigue and frustration.

Celebrating small successes and occasions helps to increase positivity and joy.

Contributing to family life, volunteering, serving, or contributing in other ways helps provide a purpose and gratification.

Support groups are an excellent way to treat mild depression, especially for those with mild memory impairment who benefit from education, insight, and comradery.

Counseling, especially Cognitive Behavioral Therapy, allows people to becomes aware of their thoughts and how they trigger certain feelings and reactions and helps adjustment with this.

Meditation has shown especially helpful in preventing the reoccurrence of depression, especially mindfulness-based cognitive therapy.

Yoga has proven to reduce stress, anxiety, and depression and also improve energy, sleep quality, and overall well-being.

Light therapy during the short, dark days of winter, or walking in the morning sun, can ease symptoms of depression sometimes after only a couple days.

Keeping a mood diary of positive things that are happening helps keep negative events in perspective. Try to make lists of activities, people, and places that increase enjoyment and schedule these things more frequently.

Smoking: There are many detrimental effects on the entire body, especially the blood vessels which supply important blood, oxygen, and nutrients to our brains. Smoking cessation is of the utmost importance to brain health. If smoking is an issue for you, don't ever quit quitting. Talk to your doctor or your local Cancer Services for assistance.

Some tips for smoking cessation per www.smokefree.gov include:

- Make a plan for a quit day

- Stay busy with things such as:

    Exercise
    Walking
    Chewing gum or hard candies
    Drinking lots of water
    Going to a movie
    Relaxing with deep breathing

- Avoid smoking triggers such as:

    Throw away cigarettes, lighters, etc.
    Avoid caffeine
    Go places where smoking isn't allowed

Achieving Your Best Brain Health with Mild Cognitive Impairment

Don't get overly fatigued, rest well
- Stay positive and reward yourself often
- Ask for help

Weight: Being overweight or obese may increase your risk of many health problems, including diabetes and heart disease. These diseases are also detrimental to the brain. Reaching and maintaining a healthy weight will help you stay heathier as you age.

Consider checking your BMI (body mass index) or check your waist size as having fat around the abdomen is found to be especially dangerous. The goal for waist size is less than 40 inches for men, and less than 35 inches for women. The goal for BMI is generally between 18.5 – 24.9. You can easily check your BMI at www.bmicalculator.org. Don't worry if you can't get to your ideal body weight. Losing even 10-15 pounds can make a huge difference.

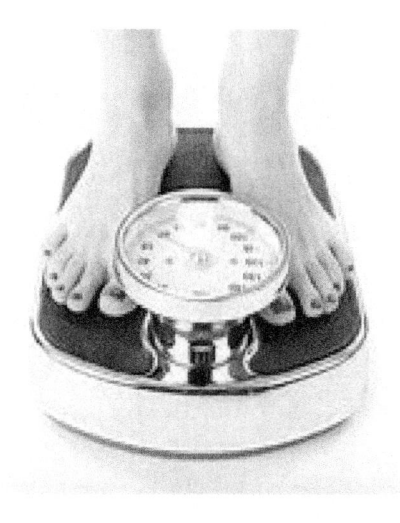

Cholesterol: It is not all "bad". Our body needs it to build cells, but too much cholesterol can cause problems. Our liver makes all the cholesterol that we need. Otherwise cholesterol comes from animal sources such as meat, poultry, and full fat dairy products.

Research suggests that healthy blood cholesterol levels may be as important for brain health as for heart health. General guidelines include the following desirable levels, however you should individualize these goals with your doctor.

- Total cholesterol: Less than 200
- Triglycerides: Less than 150
- LDL: Less than 100
- HDL for men: greater than 40
- HDL for women: greater than 50

Tips:

- Check your cholesterol and know your numbers
- Change your diet and lifestyle if necessary
- Control your cholesterol with the help from your doctor

Blood sugar: Monitoring is the main tool available to check on diabetes control for people living with diabetes. It is important for blood glucose (sugar) levels to stay in a healthy range to maintain a healthy body and brain. If blood glucose levels get too low, one can lose the ability to think and function normally. If blood sugar levels get too high and stay high, it can cause damage or complications to the body and brain over the course of many years. If you have diabetes, talk to your doctor about whether you should be checking your blood sugar levels. Blood sugar levels are individualized, however, the American Diabetes Association suggests the following targets for most adults with diabetes:

- A1C of less than 7 percent. An A1C blood test measures your average blood sugar level for the last 2 to 3 months.

- Before a meal level between 80-130mg/dl

- 1-2 hours after the beginning of a meal less than 180mg/dl

Alcohol: Current recommendations for a healthy intake of alcohol are no more than 1-2 drinks per day for a male, and no more than 1 drink per day for a woman. A "drink" is the equivalent to the following: 12 oz of beer; 5 oz of wine; or 1.5 oz of liquor, according to the Mayo clinic. There are some studies about the protective, heart healthy effects of red wine that contains resveratrols, antioxidants, and flavonoids in moderation. If alcohol is a problem for you, talk with your doctor or seek out assistance from your local Alcoholics Anonymous.

Sleep: The brain needs to be rested and re-set with at least 6-8 hours of good sleep per night. There are many articles out there that speak to the fact that you can improve your memory with a good night's sleep. We are all able to think, focus, and learn better when we are well rested.

According to the National Sleep Foundation, we need a good night's sleep to process , retain information, and to solidify memories.

Mental activity: While there is no conclusive evidence that brain exercises can slow or reverse cognitive decline, studies suggest that challenging your brain may help increase your brain activity. It is a good idea to be a "lifelong learner" and to stay curious. The activities with the most impact are those that require you to work beyond what is easy and comfortable. Trying new things is even more important and beneficial than doing the same thing, such as crosswords every day for example. Take a chance and try new things to build new brain connections such as a new language, music, lectures, courses, plays, and brain games.

Social activity: Having a strong social network can have a very positive impact on your brain and overall health. Connecting with others who are also living with cognitive changes especially can be a very comforting and satisfying experience. Connect or reconnect with friends, family, or acquaintances. Consider joining clubs, groups, senior centers, volunteering or becoming more active in church for example.

Stress: Stress causes quite significant changes in the brain which can easily affect overall cognitive ability. It is important to recognize and effectively try to deal with stress to obtain your optimal brain health. Consider certain exercises such as Meditation, Yoga or Tai-Chi. Many people will often work with a professional counselor as well with good results.

Achieving Your Best Brain Health with Mild Cognitive Impairment

Hydration: Dehydration also impacts brain function and has the ability to cause severe changes such as delirium. Ensure that you are getting at least 6-8 cups of fluid (preferably mostly water) per day. Drink caffeine minimally as it can be dehydrating. It is helpful to measure your fluid intake to see where you really are with regards to this goal. Consider carrying a water bottle with you and replacing sweetened drinks with water.

Head protection: Head trauma of any sort can lead to trouble as we age. It is important to try to prevent head trauma, especially with loss of consciousness. If you are concerned about the possibility of falling, be sure to fall proof your home and consider working with Physical Therapy. Be sure to wear your seat belt at all times, and a helmet when needed.

Regular checkups: After you have established a relationship with a physician or care provider that you trust, ensure that you are getting regular checkups. Personalize how often your visits should be with your provider.

Multivitamin: Talk to your physician to see which vitamins are a good idea for you. Be careful to avoid numerous supplements without your physician's approval.

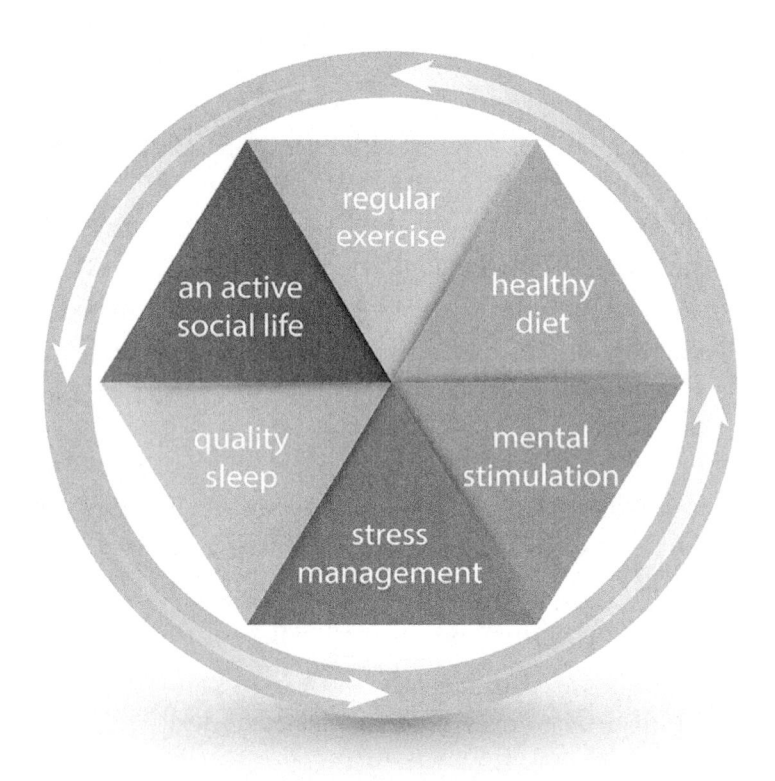

Medications to Treat Alzheimer's Disease

There are no specific medications or cures for MCI. Some doctors recommend taking medications approved for Alzheimer's disease, but research has not been able to confirm this is a good idea.

There are medications that are FDA approved for Mild, Moderate, and Severe Alzheimer's disease. These medications may help some people with cognitive and behavioral symptoms temporarily, but do not slow or stop AD. The possible benefits of these medications may help to improve a person's quality of life, ease burden to caregivers, and delay nursing home placement.

There are two different types of medications that are approved by the FDA for Alzheimer's disease. These drugs affect the activity of two different chemicals in the brain. See the table below for more details of these medications.

FDA Approved Medications for Alzheimer's Disease

Drug Name	Approved	Mild A.D.	Moderate A.D.	Severe A.D.
Acetylcholinesterase Inhibitors:				
Aricept (donepezil)	1996	X	X	X
Exelon (rivastigmine)	2000	X	X	
Razadyne (galantamine)	2001	X	X	
NMDA receptor antagonist:				
Namenda (memantine hydrochloride)	2003		X	X
Combination Therapy:				
Namzaric (memantine & donepezil)	2014		X	X
Monoclonal Antibody Therapy:				
Aduhelm (aducanumab)	2021	X		

Kari Herman

CHAPTER NINE
How Can I Prepare for My Future?

Knowledge is Power

Having a plan is the best way to ensure that the later years of your life run as smoothly as possible, and the best time to plan for your long term future is long before you need it. When it comes to your future, you will want to be the one in the driver's seat.

Communicating all of your wishes with your loved ones is also a very important part of having a plan. Planning for your long term needs is one of the smartest decisions you can make, and it is also a wonderful gift to your loved ones. By having your family up to date and on the same page, much stress will be prevented.

Making your own long term future choices now can having the following benefits:

- Creating more choices down the road
- Directing the decisions that will affect you
- Feeling less overwhelmed in the future
- Being ready to help your loved ones.

With a little bit of planning, you can create a solid foundation for the future.

Long-Term Planning

Planning for your long term future includes taking care of yourself to improve your chances for a healthy future. However there are many other things that need to be considered and planned for.

Having a master folder of all your important documents in one place that is either a fireproof locked box of safe deposit box is vital. Even better than being locked away though is open communication with your loved ones. Even those these types of topics can be uncomfortable or even painful, it is important to not ignore them. If you take the time to organize your estate and communicate your wishes, it will relieve much stress for your entire family.

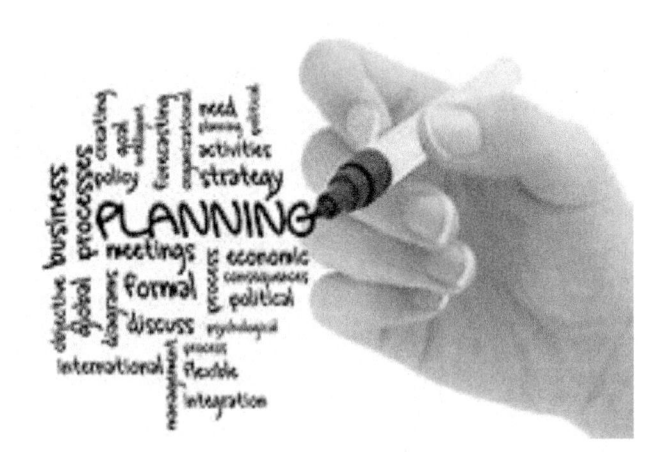

Achieving Your Best Brain Health with Mild Cognitive Impairment

Decisions About Health

Durable Power of Attorney for Healthcare: Also known as a Patient Advocate, this is the assignment of a person (or persons) selected by you to speak for you and make medical decisions for you if you become permanently or temporarily unable to make your own decisions.

This is a big decision and must not be made lightly. You will want to select someone who you feel will listen to your wishes beforehand and then follow through with honoring your wishes if the case arises. Your choice needs to be someone that you truly trust your life with.

It is important to understand that a Patient Advocate will only be your decision maker when you are not able to make your own decisions. No one can make decisions for you if you are able to make those decisions and speak for yourself. However, generally in a case of incompetence due to possible dementia or a psychiatric illness for example, your Patient Advocate will be able to make decisions on your behalf if 2 physicians determine in writing that you are unable to participate in your own healthcare decisions.

It is also important to understand that you can always change your mind about who you want to appoint.

If you have not appointed a Durable Power of Attorney for Healthcare, also known as a Patient Advocate, you are strongly encouraged to talk to one of your health care providers, consult with your local hospital, or see an attorney to do this.

Advanced Care Planning: Appointing a Patient Advocate is very important, however it is equally important that you think about and communicate your specific end of life wishes with them, so that they can honor your requests and wishes.

This will require you to really think about what matters the most to you, your values, and what your idea of meaning and quality of life is for yourself.

There are many frameworks and forms available as worksheets to help evaluate, and guide your options and decisions, for example, "Honoring Healthcare Choices".

On a basic level, different types of care and options generally fall into three categories at the end of life. This includes:

- **Life supporting** (treatment to keep you alive when your body cannot do so on it's own). This includes treatments such as CPR and ventilators

- **Life sustaining** (treatment to prolong your life when your condition cannot be reversed or cured. Tube feedings and kidney dialysis are examples of this.

- **Life enhancing** (treatments that keep you comfortable until death naturally occurs). This includes comfort measures only including pain medication for example.

While it is helpful to have a worksheet or document expressing your specific choices, it is just as important to share this with and have open communication and conversations about these details with your Patient Advocate. These forms and conversations should be reviewed and updated on a regular basis as well.

Achieving Your Best Brain Health with Mild Cognitive Impairment

These will be very personal choices and are often shaped by our own experiences with illness, injury, or death of our own loved ones.

Power of Attorney: A general Power of Attorney (POA), gives broad legal and financial powers to a person to act on your behalf. You are able to specify what powers your appointed person can have.

Durable Power of Attorney becomes immediately active upon signing and means that the POA remains active if you become mentally incompetent.

Non-Durable Power of Attorney is also immediate, but does not remain effective if you become incompetent.

Springing Power of Attorney becomes effective only when you are deemed incapacitated (e.g. A Durable Power of Attorney for Healthcare).

Wills: A will is a legal declaration of a person's wishes regarding the disposal of their property or estate after death. It goes into effect only after you pass away. A will is a public record that requires probate court involvement.

Trusts: A trust is a legal document that is frequently used in estate planning to help a person distribute or provide for a loved one after they have passed away. It is a written set of rules that determine how, what, when, and where a gift or property is to be distributed to an heir or beneficiary. A trust takes effect as soon as you create it. It can be used to begin distributing property before death, at death, or afterwards.

Other Important Decisions

Housing: Planning for your long term future gives you time to learn about services in your community and what they cost. It can also allow you to assess whether where you live now will support your changing needs as you age.

Determining where you would like to live options include:

- **Your own home**. Consider if your home will allow you to age in place. Is it able to be made handicap accessible, comfortable, and safe to age in?

- **In-home care** is a supplemental option that many people choose to be able to maintain their independence and age in place in their own homes. Care can be arranged for a few hours a week or up to 24 hours a day.

- **Assisted Living** is an option many chose. This provides a private apartment with shared meals and scheduled activities with other residents. Additional services can include transportation, housekeeping, laundry, medication assistance, assistance with bathing and dressing if needed.

- **Memory Care** is a type of assisted living for seniors that have Alzheimer's disease or dementia. It provides a secure environment with specially trained staff.

- **Skilled Nursing Homes** provide around the clock care from skilled nurses and a high level of medical care.

Achieving Your Best Brain Health with Mild Cognitive Impairment

When to Stop Driving: Ideally, the first notions and conversations about driving safety should occur long before driving becomes a problem. Early, occasional, and candid conversations with loved ones are helpful to assist monitoring and evaluate driving skills.

According to The Hartford Financial Services Group, statistics generally indicate that most older adults are safe drivers, with high safety belt use and few citations for speeding, reckless driving or alcohol-related charges. However, medical conditions, medication usage and reduced physical function can increase risk.

The topic of driving safety is often a very emotionally charged topic, due to the sense of independence that driving represents for older adults. It often leads to feelings of sadness, decreased social opportunities, and feelings of dependency on others. It is a very personal decision that must be individualized.

Ongoing discussions and objective assessments will help you as a driver and your families to evaluate the risks of your unique situation. Ongoing conversations will hopefully help you as a driver weigh decisions and agree to drive less, avoid certain road conditions, or stop driving when necessary. Ideally, the transition from driver to passenger will happen gradually over time, allowing all family members to adjust to new circumstances. Successful family conversations begin with good preparation and caring communication.

Programs such as driving safety courses, and driving skill assessments are very helpful as well for improving driving skills and recommending adaptations for safety. Warning signs for older drivers can include:

- Decreased confidence with driving
- Difficulty turning to see when backing up
- Riding the brakes
- Being easily distracted
- Having others often honk their horns at you
- Incorrect signaling
- Parking inappropriately
- Hitting curbs
- Scrapes or dents on the car, mailbox, or garage
- Failure to notice traffic signs
- Using a "copilot"
- Near misses
- Moving into the wrong lane
- Getting lost in familiar places
- Car accidents
- Failure to stop at stop signs or a red light
- Confusion about the gas and brake pedals

CONCLUSION

A diagnosis of Mild Cognitive Impairment or mild dementia can bring with it a desire to learn more, especially about how to stop or slow changes that are happening in the brain. Until there is a cure or prevention, this book attempts to give guidance and support for those living with changes or their care partners. Hopefully you have found this information useful and helpful to live your best life with changes that may be happening.

Kari Herman

REFERENCES

Alzheimer's Association. (2019). 2019 Alzheimer's Disease Facts and Figures. Retrieved from: www.alz.org

Alzheimer's Association. (4/2/2019). Alzheimer's Diagnosis, Management Improved by Brain Scans. Retrieved from: https://www.alz.org

Alzheimer's Association. (2019). Changes in Relationships. https://www.alz.org/help-support/i-have-alz/know-what-to-expect/changes-in-relationships

Alzheimer's Association. (2009). Know the 10 Signs, Early Detection Matters. Retrieved from: https://www.alz.org

Alzheimer's Association. (2019). Mild Cognitive Impairment (MCI). Retrieved from: https://www.alz.org/alzheimers-dementia/what-is-dementia/related_conditions/mild-cognitive-impairment

Alzheimer's Association. (2019). Taking Care of Yourself. Retrieved from: https://www.alz.org/help-support/i-have-alz/live-well/taking-care-of-yourself

American Association of Neurological Surgeons. (2019). Anatomy of the Brain. Retrieved from: https://www.aans.org/Patients/Neurological-Conditions-and-Treatments/Anatomy-of-the-Brain

American Diabetes Association. (2018). Checking Your Blood Glucose. Retrieved from: http://www.diabetes.org/living-with-diabetes/treatment-and-care/blood-glucose-control/checking-your-blood-glucose.html

American Diabetes Association. (2014). Diagnosing Diabetes and Learning About Prediabetes. Retrieved from: http://diabetes.org/diabetes-basics/diagnosis/

Berkely Wellness. (2014) Cholesterol & Brain Health. Retrieved from: http://www.berkeleywellness.com/healthy-mind/memory/article/cholesterol-brain-health

Boss, P. (2011). Loving Someone Who Has Dementia. San Francisco, CA: Jossey-Bass

Brainy Behavior. (2010). Aging and Role Loss. Retrieved from: http://www.brainybehavior.com/blog/2010/11/aging-and-role-loss

Center for Brain Health. (4/10/2019). Research Underscores Value of Cognitive Training for Adults with Mild Cognitive Impairment. Retrieved from: http://www.brainhealth.utdallas.edu/

Cohen. (2015). The MIND Diet: 10 Foods That Fight Alzheimer's (and 5 to Avoid). Retrieved from: https://www.cbsnews.com/media/mind-diet-foods-avoid-alzheimers-boost-brain-health/

Day, T. Wills, Trusts, POA, and Loss of Capacity. Retrieved from: https://www.longtermcarelink.net/eldercare/wills_trusts_power_of_attorney.htm

Family Caregiver Alliance National Center on Caregiving. (2011). Mild Cognitive Impairment (MCI). Retrieved from: https://www.caregiver.org/print/22291

Graff-Radford, MD. (2/2/2018). Alzheimer's: Can a Mediterranean Diet Lower My Risk?. Retrieved from: https://www.mayoclinic.org

Harvard University. (2017). What to do about Mild Cognitive Impairment. Retrieved from: https://www.health.harvard.edu/mind-and-mood/what-to-do-about-mild-cognitive-impairment

Jefferson, R. (2019). Major Clinical Trial Links High Blood Pressure and Mild Cognitive Impairment. Retrieved from: https://www.forbes.com/sites/robinseatonjefferson/2019/02/13/major-clinical-trial-links-high-blood-pressure-and-dementia-in-new-way/#16d353e5245c

Karpinski, M. (2000). The Home Care Companion's Quick Tips for Caregivers. Medford, OR: Healing Arts Communications.

Mayo Clinic. (2019). Mild Cognitive Impairment. Retrieved from: https://www.mayoclinic.org/diseases-conditions/mild-cognitive-impairment/symptoms-causes/syc-20354578?p=1

Lewis, T. (2018). Human Brain: Facts, Functions & Anatomy. Retrieved from: https://www.livescience.com/29365-human-brain.html

Mayfield Clinic Brain & Spine. (2018). Anatomy of the Brain. Retrieved from: https://mayfieldclinic.com/pe-anatbrain.htm

National Institute on Aging. (2017). Cognitive Health and Older Adults. Retrieved from: https://www.nia.nih.gov/health/cognitive-health-and-older-adults

National Institute on Aging. (2017). Planning for Long-Term Care. Retrieved from: https://www.nia.nih.gov/health/planning-long-term-care

National Institute on Aging. (2017). What is Mild Cognitive Impairment? Retrieved from: https://www.nia.nih.gov/health/what-mild-cognitive-impairment

National Institute on Aging, National Institutes of Health. (2005). Talking with Your Doctor. U.S. Department of Health and Human Services, NIH Publication No. 05-3452

National Institute of Neurological Disorders and Stroke. (2018). Know Your Brain. Retrieved from: https://www.ninds.nih.gov/disorders/Patient-Caregiver-Education/Know-Your-Brain

Newell, S. (2017). Six Tips to Prepare for Your Aging Parents' Future. Retrieved from: https://www.aegisliving.com/resource-center/six-tips-to-prepare-for-your-aging-parents-future/

Nichols, H. (2017). What Happens to the Brain as We Age? Retrieved from: https://www.medicalnewstoday.com/articles/319185.php

Peters. (2006). Ageing and the Brain. Retrieved from: https://www.ncbi.nlm.nih.gov/pmc/articles/PMC2596698

Petersen, R., Doody, R., Kurz, A., Mohs, R., Morris, J., Rabins, P., Ritchie, K.,...Winblad, B. (2001). Current Concepts in Mild Cognitive Impairment. Arch Neurol, 58.

Reinberg, S. (4/19/2019). Even a Little more Exercise might Help Your Brain Stay Young. Health Day News

Reinicke, C. (2018). If You are in your 50's, You Need to Plan for Long-Term Care Right Now. Retrieved from: https://www.cnbc.com/2018/06/22/if-youre-in-your-50s-you-need-to-plan-for-long-term-care-right-now.html

Ricon Del Rio (2016). Re-Examining "Role Loss" and Identity for Seniors. Retrieved from: https://rincondelrio.com/re-examining-role-loss-identity-seniors/

The Hartford. (February 2012). We Need to Talk...Family Conversations with Older Drivers. Hartford, CT: The Hartford Financial Services Group, Inc.

Printed in Great Britain
by Amazon